TOP FITNESS ADVICE

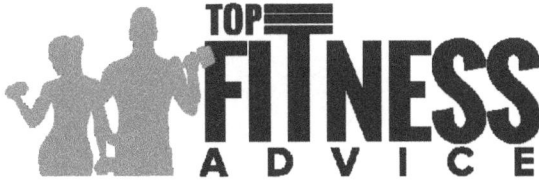

21-DAY SLIM DOWN

The 21-Day Weight Loss Guide For Beginners Wanting A Flat Belly, Firm Butt & Lean Legs (Includes Workouts, Exercises & Recipes)

Kayla Bates

ink

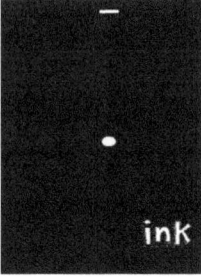

First published in 2017 by Venture Ink Publishing

Copyright © Top Fitness Advice 2019

All rights reserved.

Requests to the publisher for permission should be addressed to publishing@ventureink.co

For more information about the contents of this book or questions to the author, please contact Kayla Bates at kayla@topfitnessadvice.com

Table of Contents

Would you prefer to listen to my book, rather than read it?

Download the audiobook version for free!

If you go to the special link below and sign up to Audible as a new customer, you can get the audiobook version of my book completely free.

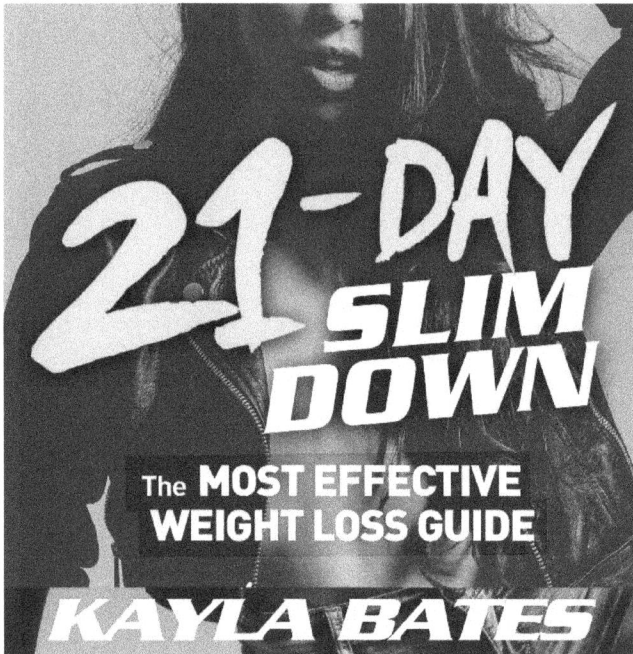

Go here to get your audiobook version for free:

TopFitnessAdvice.com/go/21Day

Who is This Book For?

This book is for anyone who wants to make a positive change in their life. Regular exercise and a good eating habit is the foundation to a happy and healthy life.

Anybody can benefit from getting into better physical shape, especially those whose jobs are not physically demanding, or have aged a few years and want a little more bounce in their step.

Any amount of exercise is better than no exercise, and coupled with a healthier eating regiment you're bound to notice an improvement in your everyday life.

This book is for anybody who is ready to accept that there are no shortcuts when it comes to fitness. Anybody ready to accept that there are no magic pills to do the job overnight and here today gone tomorrow diet fads are total garbage. There is no magic super food that can fix years of over-eating or bad dieting.

This book is for anybody who wants to truly learn how to get into better shape and is willing to put forth the effort to better themselves physically.

It's not as difficult to lose weight as magic pill commercials would have you believe it is without their product, nor is it as simple as "this one weird trick to target belly fat" complete and utter, internet clickbait, nonsense.

Some thoughts before we get into it. Pressed for time? Even if you get up for work another 10 minutes early and do some push-ups and pull ups before your morning shower, you'll already be taking steps in the right direction.

Don't want a costly gym membership? You can still do quite a few basic bodyweight exercises at home, including but not limited to push-ups, planking, pull ups (you can find pretty cheap doorframe pull up bars at your local big box store), wall squats and bench dips.

These are some pretty great exercises so don't ever feel like you won't get a return on your time investment from body weight exercises. You can even expand your home gym if you've got the real estate with a simple set of dumbbells and a decent bench. Son or daughter moved out? Got some space in the basement downstairs? Utilize this space if you refuse to go to a gym.

What Will This Book Teach You?

For the purpose of this book I will assume that the reader is new to things like tracking calories, identifying healthy alternatives to certain foods, cardio, strength training or weight loss.

My goal for this book is to teach you how to form healthier lifestyle habits and improve your overall well-being. Specifically, this book will teach you chapter by chapter about, exercise, dieting, tracking calories, and studying the results.

The goal is not to have you diet and exercise for 21 days and stop but in fact to get you interested in an active, healthier lifestyle. The 21-day challenge is just the jumpstart you need to get the ball rolling and we hope you can continue down the path to a healthier you.

I also hope to dispel some myths about weightlifting and losing weight. For example, working out does not "turn fat into muscle". If somebody claims they can turn fat into muscle, then let them know they've stumbled upon a miracle. What actually happened, was that they lost weight by eating fewer calories over an extended period of time, reducing their body fat and lifted weights progressively increasing their muscle mass.

Also, crunches won't give you abs, more likely just back pain. I recommend planking as a superior alternate exercise but keep in mind you simply must have a very small amount of body fat to have visible abs. It can be very difficult and take some pretty serious dedication to achieve that level of fitness.

Instead of killing yourself with crunches once a month, imagining yourself with a chiseled six pack, focus on the basics. Eat less food. Perform a variety of exercises. Challenge yourself with harder goals once you have actually made a foundation for a fitter lifestyle.

That's it. No secrets, no "one weird trick", no magic pills. Just adjusting eating habits, limiting calorie intake over time and lifting weights.

Of course, some people have health complications or medication that affects their weight. I won't pretend to know how to help people under these circumstances, other than recommend they talk to their family doctor or a dietician.

The reason there is so much nonsense advertising and misinformation floating around when it comes to exercise and weight loss is simple; it's more comforting to imagine an easy solution you just haven't found yet rather than tracking every meal and lifting weights or exercising regularly.

So many people use this desire for an easy out to promote their own magic substance to bolster sales or craft clickbait. Click bait is any attention-grabbing headline to draw you to click on an ad.

"Lose belly fat with this one weird trick" type of nonsense comes to mind when thinking about click bait. Why does this exist? To get you on a webpage where whoever owns the web page is being paid for all the views of ads that their website contains or is trying to sell you something.

Think about it like this, if there really was an easy, fast, magic solution to get in shape, you probably wouldn't stumble across it on a random webpage ad, redirecting you to a questionable website.

In fact, if such a product existed, it would probably sell billions and be in the news headlines for months to come.

Another way to spot this nonsense is to know that you literally cannot target which parts of your body you want to burn fat on. Arm curls don't burn arm fat and running doesn't burn leg fat.

Weight loss is a whole-body thing and you have no control over what fat gets burning priority over the other parts. If you're not satisfied with how much belly fat you've burned so far, you simply have to keep on hitting your calorie goals till you're happy with that area.

In summary, ideally, you will learn how to set calorie goals, how to track progress, the different ways of tracking progress, how to track calories, how to track exercise goals, establish a regular exercise schedule, learn the basics of weightlifting, learn proper form for the primary lifts, set lift goals, understand cheat days, avoid wasting time on "shortcuts" and how to generally become more fit.

Introduction to the 21-day Fitness Challenge

Intro to Exercising

Now it is true that certain exercises will burn more calories than others but burning enough calories is much, much harder than tracking your calorie intake and not exceeding your limit for the day.

I actually find it more difficult to eat within my calorie goal when burning calories. That may sound confusing, but we'll talk about that more later on when we talk about cardio and weight loss.

Whether you plan on lifting weights at your local gym, running on the treadmill at home or simply going for a walk once a day this book can help you reach your fitness goals, though I personally recommend weight lifting.

Now what's the hardest part about exercising?

Personally, I would say the hardest part is getting into the rhythm of things. Establishing an exercise schedule and sticking to it. It does not matter if you lift weights, swim, bike, run or walk, so long as you get some form of physical activity in during the day where you can measure progress and results.

Once you have decided on a measurable activity you can begin establishing a schedule. For example, let's say you decide to start lifting weights at the gym, 3 times per week. Great! Now let's say you want to bench press on Mondays, deadlift on Wednesdays and squat on Fridays.

Plan is looking pretty good so far but be careful not to overdo it at the gym, especially if it's been a while or you are newcomer to weightlifting. Forewarning, you will be sore when you wake up the next morning. In fact, your muscles will probably ache worse than you have ever felt previously. You will initially hate this feeling but trust me, you will learn to love it as it means you are putting on muscle and getting healthier.

Note: you should be SORE not in PAIN, there is a very distinct difference. If you're are hurting or in pain you need to either, ask somebody who works at your gym how to properly perform these lifts or watch some video guides online.

Now's a good time to dispel a common myth about weightlifting for women. If you are a female and you lift weights you will not magically transform into a musclebound monster and lose your petite form overnight.

You will however get stronger and more defined muscles. If you do not wish to look like models on sports supplement containers, have no fear, as that would take years of serious dedication to achieve that look.

Now back to your exercise plan, you are typically going to perform 3 "sets" of 5-8 "reps". "Sets" are how many times you plan on performing each set of 5-8 "reps" and reps are how many times you lift that weight for the complete motion of that particular exercise.

For example, you want to do 3 sets of 5-8 reps so you need to figure how much weight you lift at least 5 times but not more than 8, then repeat that exercise for a total of 3 times.

Typically, you're first set is a warm up set and will be the lightest weight, gradually adding weight per set. The sets after your warm up set are your working sets. And I don't usually count the warm up set as one of my 3-4 sets.

Before we move on to dieting and tracking, a few pieces of advice. Nobody at the gym is judging you because you are a newcomer; in fact, most gym regulars and staff would much prefer to help show a newcomer the ropes rather than see someone injure themselves.

Additionally, do yourself a favor and bring some running shoes (flat bottom shoes if you plan on squatting or deadlifting) and a reusable bottle for water.

Let's take a moment to talk about supplements. You do not have to take pre-workout, creatine, protein powder, fish oil pills, green tea extract or any one of the hundreds of workout supplements available on the market. They are marketed as an exercise aid in pill or powder form.

These are expensive supplements and most importantly they are completely optional. If you want to try one or more of them in combination with healthy workout regime, that's entirely your choice. You are by no means doomed to fail without these pills and powders.

Just a thought, all these supplements claim to aid in conjunction with regular exercise. Wonder why they all say that, eh. Probably because they don't do much of anything and hope results from actually working out and dieting mask that fact and you tell yourself it was their product.

Now that we have got somewhat of an idea what our 21 days of exercising is going to look like and have got a few key tips to keep in mind, we can start talking about something not many people are too keen on: Dieting. I think what I have to say about dieting will give you a new perspective.

Intro to Dieting

Believe it or not, dieting is not nearly as scary as people would often have you believe. The key to dieting is tracking everything you eat during the course of the day and making sure you don't exceed your caloric limit for the day.

Now, why does dieting complement exercise so well?

Think about it like putting defined muscle in the space where fat used to show the most. It's kind of like reshaping your body, the way a sculptor molds clay. You could say losing fat is equally as important to gaining muscle, when it comes to getting a fitter body.

My personal favourite app for this is MyFitnessPal. Now I know how incredibly inconvenient it sounds to have to track every single thing you eat over the course of a busy day, but trust me, it's really not that bad. In fact, many apps allow you to use your camera on your smartphone as a barcode reader and you can scan your meals right into your app before your meal.

The only real inconvenience I have found with tracking calories is the time it takes to add together all the individual ingredients in recipes for home cooked meals. However, you only have to do this once and you can generally save your custom meals into the app.

Once you get a steady rhythm of logging your meals and recording your weight for the day you will absolutely start to see results. The app only takes a few minutes to set up and you only need to enter your height, weight, gender, age and average activity level for the day to start figuring out how many calories you can eat in a day while still losing weight.

Same goes for bulking up (intentional weight gain) but with a minimum calorie goal for the day rather than a maximum. That being you still want to hit your goal number, not extremely under or over it.

You pick all of your own exercises, meals and make your own goals and the app gives you the calorie number you need to reach these goals. It even gives you a little added motivation at the end of each day when you finish logging giving you a projection of how much you would weigh if every day was like that day.

The more you use the app and follow your calorie goals the easier it gets. Before you know it, you'll be 20 pounds' lighter and find yourself with a much smaller appetite.

The first week of tracking what you put into your body is a real eye opener. It's crazy to see how many calories are in certain foods, like muffins for example, around 400 or so. Now your initial weight loss will be the most significant as you shed pounds you will need to eat fewer calories.

Personally, I like to weight myself every morning before my shower but be warned, the scale can be misleading. If you're lifting weights and putting on some muscle you may not see as much weight loss as if you had only dieted.

Now with that being said if you just want to get smaller, eating fewer calories is the single most important factor. There are other ways to measure weight loss, but we'll get into those later.

Cardio can be a part of an active healthy lifestyle but you will never outrun a bad diet. It is simply far easier to just avoid eating that muffin than trying to burn off those 400 calories on a treadmill.

Tips and Tricks

Some important tips: Expect some pretty significant fluctuations in your weight from day to day. Depending on how much water you've drank, how many meals, what you had for those meals and what clothes you're wearing you can expect your weight to easily vary by 5 or more pounds.

Another tip, try and take your weight everyday around the same time and with as few variables as possible. I find the easiest way to do this is to wake up in the morning and before showering, take your weight. No clothes and weighing yourself around the same time every day is about as consistent as is possible.

Also, good to note, try to avoid wasting your calories whenever possible. Sugary snacks, salty junk food and alcohol will leave you feeling hungry anyway and you'll have fewer calories to spend on foods high in protein and fat.

Real meals, especially home cooked, foods high in protein and fat will keep you feeling fuller, longer than the same number of calories from junky foods would.

Drinking your calories is quite possibly the fastest way to burn through your daily allotment. Sugary soda and juices will burn up your calories before your eyes and leaving you feeling unsatisfied and still hungry.

Possibly the most important piece of advice I can give for dieting is to focus on the actual number of calories you took in for that day. While it is true eating cookies all day but still eating within your goal will still result in weight loss, it's not exactly the healthiest way to go about it.

Use your common sense when deciding what to eat that day. You don't have to cut out your favourite meals and you can still snack at any time of the day. Just remember to keep it within your calorie goal, get plenty of sleep, and keep your proportions sensible.

Let's take a moment to dispel a common myth about dieting. You do not need to do cardio to lose weight. I personally actually find cardio makes sticking to my calorie limit for the day more difficult. My appetite goes crazy after a bout of cardio training and I usually end up eating far more calories than I have burned off.

Cardio is great for mostly one thing, and that's getting better at cardio. Now with that said cardio is still a great and healthy activity but not mandatory for weight loss.

In fact, if you are truly so busy during every day you have no time to exercise whatsoever you can still lose weight. Just change you weight loss app activity level to "little to no activity during the day".

Keep in mind the less active you are during the day the lower your overall allotment for calories per day will be. This shouldn't necessarily make it harder to lose weight as your appetite shouldn't be too difficult to manage on days when you're not physically active.

One final point to make about dieting before we move on to tracking, is cheat days. What are they and how often should you take them?

Cheat days are days when you ignore your current diet. They are not inherently good or bad as they are tricky to manage.

This sounds counter intuitive but sometimes you just want to go out the bar with your friends and eat junk food or stay at home and eat a pizza to yourself. We're all only human and inevitably get these urges to cheat on our diets.

Cheat days are fine to take once in a while as your body weight is reflection of your average calorie intake. If I had to set a limit on cheat days, I would say no more than 2 cheat days per month.

Why should you take cheat days? A good diet is important but it shouldn't overly interfere with other aspects of your life, like avoiding going out for lunch or drinks with your friends.

Moderation is key and diet is no exception. Don't waste all your calories on empty booze calories but don't stress yourself out over being surgically precise with your calories every single day. A good diet should be part of your life, not all of it.

Now that we've got a decent grasp on dieting let's look at my favourite part of this whole thing: tracking.

Intro to Tracking

Now, why is tracking my favourite part of this whole thing? Because it's measurable progress. Its results you can look at objectively and compare them with your starting baseline. Basically, its gratification for the work you put it. So, how do you measure your progress? It entirely depends on what you chose for your goal!

Weight loss is probably the most difficult to measure as it has many factors. If weight loss was your goal, make sure to not only look at the numbers on the scale; but to also take waist measurements, before and after photos, and neck measurements.

You especially want to measure more than just your weight if you plan on weightlifting as well as dieting. Don't get discouraged by numbers on scale when you could very well be adding muscle to your weight.

However, do not use this logic as a crutch for not losing weight, you have to actually take these measurements. Don't just assume extra muscle is the culprit of your less than expected weight loss.

Weightlifting is probably the easiest thing to measure and track as all the weights are labeled and exercises are broken into sets and reps.

If you plan on performing some off the most important exercises, bench press, deadlift, and squat, you will also want to record your personal records(PRs) for these lifts. Spend more than 2 seconds in any gym and you're likely to hear gym buddies discussing their max bench, squat or deadlift. This simply means the most weight you can perform for a single repetition.

There are countless apps for your smartphone you can use to track your weightlifting progress, in fact MyFitnessPal can do it.

Of course, you always just bring a pad and pen to the gym too. What matters is that you're tracking your lifts because between work, social life and the variety of exercises possible, you will forget these numbers otherwise.

Here's a pretty basic example of what your exercise tracking should look like:

Monday – Chest: Barbell Bench Press

- Set 1: 100 x 8
- Set 2: 120 x 7

- Set 3: 140 x 6
- PR 165 x 1

Tuesday – Back: Barbell Deadlifts

- Set 1: 135 x 8
- Set 2: 155 x 8
- Set 3: 175 x 5
- PR 200 x 1

Friday – Legs: Barbell Squats

- Set 1: 135 x 7
- Set 2: 145 x 6
- Set 3: 175 x 5
- PR 200 x 1

Notes

- Read "45 x 8" as forty-five pounds being lifted for 8 repetitions

- The weight here is for example purposes only, start with the bar only to get a feel for the motion and slowly add weight

- Only attempt PRs once you're more familiar with the lifts

- Always have a spotter (another person who can help you lift the weight should you fail your rep attempt)

- Always engage the safeties (adjustable metals bar attached to the equipment designed to stop the weight from coming down too far if you fail the lift)

- Deadlifts require no spotter or safeties – watch video guides online and do some research before attempting this

This is about as simple as a workout regime can get yet still focuses on the three most popular muscle and strength building lifts. It's an easy format for newcomers to get familiar with but still allows for more exercises and/or training days to be added.

Now that we've got the absolute basics of exercise, diet and tracking nailed down we can start we can start on week 1 of the challenge.

Not every day has to be a PR attempt day, in fact lifting heavy for one rep isn't even necessary, it's just another way of exercising. Although it does make for a good reference point when figuring out how much weight you should be lifting but more on that later.

I hope that you are enjoying this book so far, and if you could spare 30 seconds, I would greatly appreciate you leaving a review on Amazon.com.

Are You ALWAYS Hungry When You Try to Lose Weight?

Discover How to STOP Starving Yourself & Lose Weight FASTER By Eating MORE Food!

For this month only, you can get Kayla's best-selling & most popular book absolutely free – *The Ultimate Guide to Healthy Eating & Losing Weight Without Starving Yourself!*

Get Your FREE Copy Here:
TopFitnessAdvice.com/Book

Discover how you can **start eating MORE food** and see weight loss results faster than ever before. Learn about the 10 most powerful fat-burning foods and how they boost the rate that your body burns fat. And last but not least, finally put an end to your emotional or "bored" eating habits. With this book, readers were able to significantly improve their weight loss results. So, it's highly recommended that you get this book, especially while it's free!

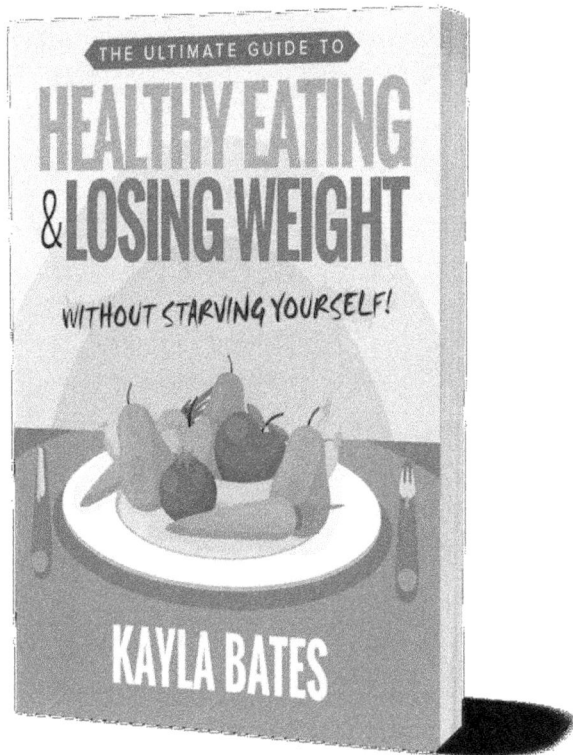

Get Your FREE Copy Here:

TopFitnessAdvice.com/Book

Week 1

Total Overhaul

Dieting Week 1

The first step to a truly successful change in diet is to change the way you think about food. Once you start logging every piece of food in your tracking app you will quickly realize why this is necessary.

You have to look at food the same way you would look at your budget. You only have a finite number of calories to spend.

Sure, you can waste them on junk you don't need, but in the same way wasting money on stuff you didn't need only provides the briefest of satisfaction and you won't have enough coin to spend on more fulfilling things.

Your first week of dieting should be a total eye-opener to just how much you overspend your calories. It's so easy to just not remember how many little things you snacked on that day, but they all add up and tracking it all will keep you honest.

Let's talk about the most important changes you can make to start off with for meal and snack habits.

For breakfast, avoid juices like apple and orange juice. They have similar amounts of sugar and calories as soda and do nothing to keep you feeling full.

Think about eating one or two pieces of turkey bacon and one or two eggs with a single slice of toast. Sounds like a lot of calories but for the packages I scanned, it only adds up to about 400 calories. 100 for both slices of bacon, 180 for both eggs and 110 for the toast. The same as a single pumpkin spice muffin from Tim Horton's.

Of course, all brands and variations on foods will yield different calorie values but these days there are tons of low calorie options.

Substitute ground beef with ground turkey, drink diet soda if you must have soda, buy real cheese in single slice form, snack on carrots rather than chips and dip.

Once you find the meal options that work best for you, try to plan your meals out so they're spread out over the course of the day. It's easier to stick to your diet if your calories are spread out into three balanced meals, with a light snack in between, over the course of the days as opposed to spending them all in one sitting on an appetizer, entrée and dessert.

All About Dieting

Another misconception about dieting is that you can no longer go out to lunch with your friends or eat fast food. It all depends on what you order.

Obviously home cooked meals are better, for about every reason you can think of, but you also don't have to avoid eating at restaurants and fast food places like the plague.

If you're eating fast food, think about what you're ordering in terms of calories. A greasy double cheese burger full flavour sauces is obviously going to be costly, so try and order a grilled chicken sandwich.

Best advice I can give is to find the restaurant in your calorie tracking app and order what fits your calorie budget.

Some foods may surprise you, like salads for example. Depending on the fast food place and the type of salad you could easily be looking at the same calorie count as a burger.

Luckily, the app I use to track my calories easily finds fast food menu items so recording them is usually no problem. The only time eating out causes some issues with accurately tracking calories is when you eat at smaller or family run restaurants that aren't in your apps database.

What I do in this situation is look for a well-known chair restaurant that offers a similar item. Odds are there will be something close enough in the database and close enough is better than not logging anything at all.

An important thing to learn early on in your diet; healthy does not equal low calorie and just because something is low in calories doesn't make it healthy.

Avocado, for example, considered to be a health food. It's also relatively high in calories. Should you strip them from your diet? Absolutely not. Should you eat them in moderation? Absolutely.

The key is not to fall into a mindset where you tell yourself, "dieting is so hard but I'm still going to stick to a super strict diet even though it sucks and I'll be hungry all the time and I have to give up the tasty food in my life".

Dieting should be about realizing how many calories your body should be getting in a day and how many you are really putting into your body. You don't have to survive on blended vegetables for the rest of your life to lose weight, you just have to make an effort to more reasonable portions.

Some Final Tips for Total Overhaul Week 1:

- Portion control, use a smaller plate, weigh your food, follow the serving size recommended.

- Be patient, don't expect to shed 20 pounds your first week.

- The longer you keep up the new diet the more under control your appetite will get.

- Alcohol has a shocking number of calories, especially mixed specialty drinks – shot of whiskey: 105 calories, margarita: 270 calories.

- Alcohol is a combination of no nutritional value, drinking your calories, and failing to satisfy your hunger.

- Save cheat days for drinking and partying.

The first week of overhauling your diet will undoubtedly be the hardest part of your reshaping you're eating habits permanently. Meaning it only gets easier from here as you start shedding a few pounds and get you appetite under control.

Losing weight is awesome but you know what's even better? Putting on some muscle after the weights gone.

It's one thing to get smaller, but seeing muscle definition where there used to be fat? It's got to be one of the best feelings ever, especially when you compare before and after pictures.

We'll talk more about progress pictures later, but just know that seeing muscle definition is one of the most motivating things there is. Second only to see the scale move in the right direction, if you've ever struggled with your weight.

Exercising Week 1

Weight loss is exactly what it sounds like; lose weight and you'll just get smaller and leaner.

If you want to look more muscular you'll need to do some form of exercise, whether it be weightlifting (my personal favourite and probably the easiest thing to pick up relatively quickly if your typically pretty sediment) or swimming, or playing hockey.

Weightlifting is great for several reasons. The first reason being that I don't find it to burn many calories. Sounds crazy, right?

I actually prefer exercises that don't burn many calories (makes me hungry after the workout and harder to keep under my calorie goal) and are more focused on strength training. The reasoning behind this is that I prefer to build muscle and get stronger as I follow my calorie tracking goals to lose fat and build up muscle so I'm not only leaner, but now have a more muscular build.

The second reason weightlifting is great is because it's incredibly easy to track your progress and set goals, and we all know how important reaching goals is. It allows us to feel some additional gratification when we hit that new bench press one rep max. Its results for the work we put in.

The last reason weightlifting is great is simply all the health benefits that follow. Aside from the pretty major things like increasing muscle mass instead of gradually losing it over time, the little things it adds to are very appreciable. Not being out of breath from climbing the stairs at home feels better than sore muscles ache.

It's not all rainbows and sunshine though because you will be sore. In fact, if you've never lifted weights before you will probably be so sore that quitting will be very appealing.

Remember what I said earlier though because I can't say it enough. You will learn to love this feeling and will gradually get less sore. After a few weeks, you can expect to see some pretty awesome things start to happen, especially if you've been losing weight.

We've already mentioned some basic exercises for the major muscle groups but let me recommend some other lifts for smaller muscles. Everybody loves to train biceps and triceps.

The feeling of your arms getting pumped up during a good training session is addictive.

The Specifics

For biceps, I recommend standing alternating dumbbell curls:

1. Grab two dumbbells of the same weight and take a stance where your feet are shoulder width apart.

2. Hold the dumbbells so that your palms are facing your legs.

3. Lift one of the weights upwards while gradually turning your hands 90 degrees until your palm is facing upwards.

4. Hold the weight here for just a second and feel the squeeze in your bicep.

5. Slowly and in a controlled manner, lower the weight back to the starting position turning your palm to face your leg once again.

6. Repeat this for the other arm.

Note that your elbow should not move from your side. Your elbow should remain stationary as your forearm raises.

If you do not plan on going to your local gym, I recommend buying a half decent chin up bar for your doorframe.

Chin-ups are excellent for biceps and also work your upper back. I strongly recommend not getting the kind which is just a straight bar that extends across the gap in your doorway, but rather the kind the pushes against the wall above the moulding.

Alternatively, you can buy some dumbbells. Start with 15 lbs or so and move up to 30 lbs. If you find yourself needing heavier weights, it may be time to invest in a gym membership.

For triceps, I recommend one arm cable pulldowns:

1. Start by attaching the handle attachment for one arm exercises.

2. Raise the cable to the highest position and stand directly in front of the handle.

3. Adopt a shoulder width stance with the cable in the middle of your stance.

4. Grab the handle with your palm facing upwards.

5. Slowly pull the handle downwards, while keeping your elbow at your side, until your forearm is straight out and making a 90-degree angle with your upper arm. You're now in the starting position.

6. Slowly turn your palm towards your leg as you fully extend your arm and your palm is now facing your leg.

7. Hold this for just a moment and feel the squeeze in your triceps.

8. Return to the starting position slowly and repeat.

Alternatively, you can find a chair and table and perform bench dips:

1. Line up a chair and a short table.

2. Grab the edge of your seat and bridge the gap with your legs.

3. Slowly lower yourself down until your arms make a 90-degree angle and raise yourself back up.

4. Your feet should remain still while the rest of your body dips down.

Note that your elbows should remain at your side. Push-ups are another great triceps exercise though they mostly work your chest.

These are just some of my personal favourites. There are so many resources online for finding new lifts, don't be scared to try some others!

Results Week 1

Let's tally up what we've got so far. One week of exercise, and one week of tracking our calories. The scale probably hasn't moved very much and you are probably pretty sore right about now, cursing this 21- Day Fitness Challenge. It would only be of concern if you did not feel this way. Like I said earlier, getting into a rhythm and adjusting to it is going to be the hardest part.

The scale not budging and your lifts seeming weak are the least important thing to be on your mind right now. The only thing you should be thinking about right now is that you are actually taking steps in the right direction. The kind of steps that are not easy to take, but the steps you will look back on and be unendingly grateful that you took them at all.

It will get easier. This is what I wish I knew when I started. More importantly, exercise and tracking calories will become part of your everyday life. You'll know you've made it when doing this doesn't even cross your mind as something of note for the day.

If the scale moves, up or down, record that in your app. I prefer MyFitnessPal for this as I can update my weight over time and see a graph of ups and downs but an overall declining line over time.

Don't post about going to the gym to social media, don't brag about your new diet to your friends, don't even tell anybody unless they ask. Don't make a big deal about anything because you don't yet have enough results. Don't do anything besides record what weight you lifted and what your weight is, and keep on tracking calories.

Telling people, you are tracking your calories and making social media posts about your goals does not give you accountability, it gives you a temporary degree of satisfaction for results you have not yet achieved.

Anybody can track their calories for a week, post it to Facebook and quit. The only thing you'll hear about is questions whether or not you're still working out or dieting.

Real feedback on your results happens not when you tell other people that you've been hitting the gym or dieting, but when others tell you that you look leaner, more muscular.

The Truth

This is going to take so much longer than 21 days, and like I said in the beginning, that's not the point of this challenge. That's why it's so important to not make big deal about results or seeming lack of; there's nothing to be upset about.

To reiterate, the point of this challenge is to get you to see that there is no secret to fitness. Lift, track, study results and repeat. Use these 21 days as the format to follow for months to come.

If you only ever have your mind on results and can't fathom following this format for months or even a year or two, you've not yet made these habits a non-noteworthy part of your everyday life.

Don't let the first week discourage you. In fact, you should congratulate yourself on actually making a change. It's so easy to make a New Year's resolution claiming to lose weight or get in shape. Always easier said than done and here you are, doing, not saying.

That being said this is hardest point in making these changes. This is when you're going to be the sorest, lifting the least weight, making the most mistakes, and seeing the least weight loss. Keep that in mind when you're reviewing your results.

Keeps things in perspective.

Once again, thank you for reading this book, and I hope you're getting a lot of valuable information. I would greatly appreciate it if you could take 30 seconds to leave me a review for this book on Amazon.com.

Enjoying this book?

Check out my other best sellers!

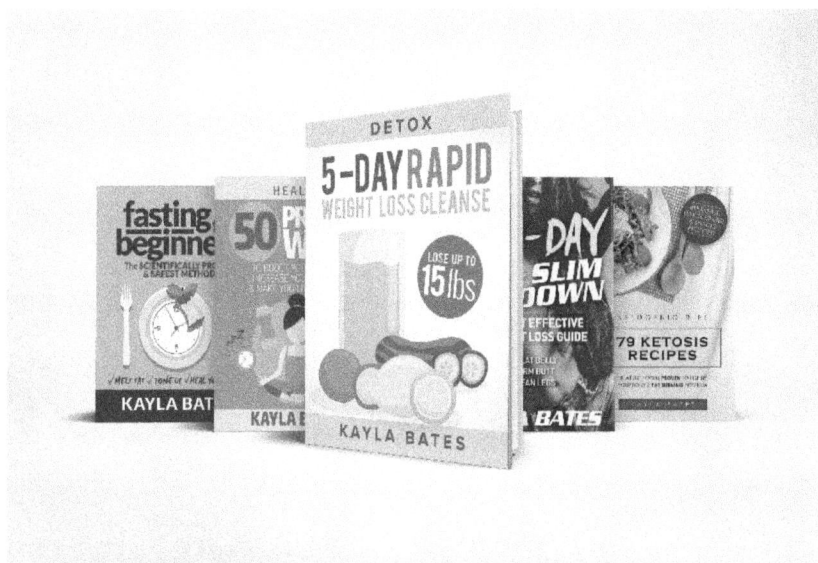

Get your next book on sale here:

TopFitnessAdvice.com/go/Kayla

Adjusting and Refining

Dieting week 2

If you've made it this far, there's not too many valid reasons to give up now. May as well keep going forward to see what kind of results lie ahead in the future.

By now I imagine you've got the hang of things to some degree. Sure, you'll still discover the odd food that surprises you calorically, but you'll likely have an understanding of what a good balanced number of calories over the course of a day should like in meal form.

I'm sure, if you took my advice, you're finding MyFitnessPal to be an excellent tracking app. The fact that once you scan and enter a particular item, it stays in your recent foods is pretty awesome.

Once you've got a pretty healthy database of foods entered you won't even have to scan nearly as often. Just scroll down through your recent foods and select the item and quantity. Some foods can be tricky to get the quantity right so either guess or pick up a cheap food scale.

I should also mention that if you are struggling with finding appropriate foods to be eating, it may be time to start planning meals. I don't personally find this to be all that important, but I know it helps some people and I think I know why.

When you're going about your day, assuming you're pretty busy with life and work, I can see how reading the labels on your food gets to the bottom of your priority list.

This is where meal planning comes in handy. If you've only got free time after work or on the weekends you can use this time to plan out your meals for the following week(s).

Taking a lunch to work/school/college is not only good for time and calorie management, it also saves you money. The way I would do this is to look up some low-calorie lunch recipes and buy all the ingredients, or just scan what I have around the house for the things that I typically eat for lunch. Get some meal ideas and input them into your tracking app.

If you're really strapped for time you can even go as far to enter the meals into your tracking app for days in the future. Now all you have to do is make sure the right meal for that day is in the fridge for you to take to work in the morning.

All you have to do is refer to your tracking app, tap over to the right day for that week and see what you have planned out. I'd also make sure to scan all of the ingredients for, a sandwich let's say, as I'm throwing it together.

If you're cooking a large quantity of food, pick out what you want for the week and either freeze the rest or serve the rest to anybody else whose home during lunch; they can take some of your food for work/school/college lunch too. Don't forget that you can use MyFitnessPal to make custom food entries. You'll only have to figure out the calories for each recipe once.

It's a little tricky to add custom foods so I'll walk you through it. The first thing I would do is pick a meal on a day where you have no other entries. Let's say under the dinner section. Scan each individual ingredient and make sure you've got the right quantities figured out. Grab the total for all these and write it down.

Now when you create a custom food you just have to name it, pick the serving size (in grams or cups), and how many servings you had and how many calories are in it.

I wouldn't bother with all the other nutritional information. That info is still important but not really for just pure weight loss. Remember were tracking calories, not carbs and fats. I find tracking all that to be way too much work. Besides, calories are what determine weight loss.

Tupperware containers are your best friends when it comes to meal planning.

You can freeze different meals in them for different days of the week, use it to bring your food into work, and you can't over eat more than the serving that you divvied up for that day because the rest is frozen and at home.

Another thing I'm sure you've noticed by now is that "health" and "breakfast" bars aren't really so healthy or keep you full as much as a proper breakfast. No shortcuts, remember?

I suppose it's better than skipping breakfast altogether but try to at least pick one food that is high in protein and fat to keep you feeling fuller for a longer period of time.

If you're finding you just don't have time for breakfast, you could make up a bagel or some kind of remotely decent breakfast item the night before and stick it in your fridge.

Exercising Week Two

Hopefully you haven't convinced yourself weightlifting isn't for you by now, because that simply isn't true.

I promise you if you stick it out for a couple of weeks you will be less and less sore after your time at the gym. You can also expect to see you're most significant gains start happening early into your weightlifting hobby.

What could be a better, more enriching hobby than weightlifting? You meet new people, get stronger, gain more muscle mass and generally set and meet your own personal goals. You will also reap all of the health benefits that follow.

But maybe you absolutely have fallen in love with bench press but hate push-ups. That's fine, in fact it's normal to favor some lifts over others. There are so many different exercises that you can try, and you won't like all of them.

You may find some are hard on your joints or the lift simply isn't hitting your muscles like you want it to. I can pretty much guarantee you can find an alternative exercise for the muscle group that you want to work on.

My personal favourite online resource for checking form and finding new exercises to perform is bodybuilding.com. They also sell just about any supplement under the sun, but you already know my opinion on those. I like to pick a muscle group and sort by ratings and see what exercises get the best reviews from people. They also have step by step videos to explain exactly how to safely lift the weight. This is an indispensable resource when it comes to finding new lifts and performing them safely.

Improper weight lifting can cause major injury and even death so it is very important to make sure you are doing things properly.

If you are new to an exercise it is never a bad idea to start off with low weight until you get used to the weight lifting technique and the movement of the exercise.

I'm sure by now you've realized that nobody at the gym is watching you or cares about how much weight you're lifting. People go to the gym for different reasons but none of those reasons are to judge the other people there.

You should never feel self-conscious at the gym because we all have good and bad gym days and we all look different.

Judging an overweight person at the gym is like judging a broke person establishing a spending budget. I can also pretty much guarantee any half decent gym will not tolerate bullying in any form.

Exercise Goals

Let's talk about specific exercise goals.

Goals can come in all shapes and sizes and have all different lengths of time for the end goal to be met. Some people want get lean and defined and some people want to get as much mass as possible. It's actually pretty straightforward.

If you want to get more muscle definition, you have to decrease your body fat. You can measure your body fat percentage with a kit from bodybuilding.com or you can ask your dietician/family doctor to find out for you.

The simplest way to measure your body fat is with the kit. It works by using a pair of calipers to measure the indicated parts of your body and figuring out your total percentage on the included chart.

Strong and lean builds is typically where you'll find swimmers, cyclists and runners. People who are pretty light, thin but have plenty of endurance.

If you want to train for size, you're going to need to eat and lift. A lot. If you look at any strong man competition, you'll notice the lifters are very bulky. No doubt they train hard and workout a ton but they will look husky. This is more for people who want to lift Atlas stones rather than look good at the beach.

This is where you see the husky guy at the gym in a sweater whose bench pressing 400lbs. They aren't usually very defined, but are big and strong. They tend to focus on bench press, squats and deadlifts, and you likely won't seem them on the treadmill.

Then there's my personal favourite training ideology: bodybuilding. Lifting weights at the gym for bigger muscles and dieting to lower body fat. It's a nicely balanced training method. You'll get bigger, more definition and improve your health.

There's a common myth that you want to lift for many reps to get more defined, and to lift fewer reps for mass. The size bit mostly comes from your diet. The best set and rep range I would recommend for anybody is to lift 3-4 sets for 5-8 reps.

The most important thing to keep in mind is that any form of exercise and diet will make you stronger and healthier.

Of course, that was a pretty hasty generalization of those exercise ideologies and that's because I don't want you to overthink what you're doing and distract yourself from your basic fitness goals. It would take far too long to go into serious depth about these activities. Not to mention this is just supposed to be a basic starting point to introduce you to fitness.

For the purpose of this challenge I strongly recommend focusing on the main lifts, bench press, dead lifts, and squats, for 3-4 sets and 5-8 reps.

Make these the foundation of your fitness goals and branch out from there if you feel the desire. I would hazard to say there's as much useful information on the internet about each specific activity as there is exercise myths.

Some Tips

- Search for alternative exercises for the same muscle groups on the internet.

- Avoid the leg extension machine and the smith machine; they force you to adjust to the movement rather than adjusting to fit your movement.

- Load up your favourite music on your phone and bring decent headphones; wireless is recommended.

- Rest days are just as important as lift days; limit training to 5 days a week.

Results Week 2

Well here you are. You have officially survived two weeks of being active and eating better.

You have a little bit more data to look at in your tracking app, not enough for timeline, but you can start to see how these results make a neat little weight loss graph. Remember you can track more than just weight loss with most apps too.

Some prefer to track their waist, neck or hip measurements as opposed to their weight. This is an excellent way to track results if you're concerned about added muscle throwing off your perception of weight loss.

It's also more consistent as we've already discussed that your weight has many variables, whereas your neck, hips and waist won't. It's also never a bad idea to take progress pictures. I know it can feel embarrassing to take a picture of yourself when you're not exactly happy with how your body currently looks, but you will regret not taking pictures after you lose some weight.

Weight loss is so gradual, it's easy to get dissuaded by the apparent lack of results. When you have a starting reference point for comparison a few weeks down the road, it becomes much more obvious the difference you have made to your body.

Progress pictures can also serve as a way to remind yourself why being active and eating reasonably is so important. After you've lost weight you can look back to your starting picturing for motivation to keep going.

Progress pictures are also an amazing way to see the changes in your muscle definition. When done right, progress pictures can show the body fat loss around your arms, thighs, belly, hips, waist and face. It shows how your body tightens up and you can see how your muscles start to outline and stand out more.

If you do decide to take progress pictures, which I highly recommend, this is the right way to do it:

- Before you endeavor on any weight loss, find a decent size mirror where you can get a picture of most of your body.

- You'll want to strip down to at least your underwear and take a picture straight on and a side portrait. It never hurts to take a close up shot of your face as well so you can see how weight loss narrows down your face and neck.

- Also, make sure the lighting is consistent for all of your pictures. It can be tricky getting consistent shots and lighting is key. People often abuse lighting for pictures to make themselves look more toned. You're only lying to yourself if you do this.

- Another thing is to make a note of the date you took the picture so you can easily line them all up after a few weeks/months and see the changes over a timeline.

I'm not sure about other tracking apps but I know that MyFitnessPal allows you to take progress pictures under the "progress" tab.

I recommend doing this because you can update your weight for the day and connect a progress picture with it. A picture is worth a thousand words and all that, I suppose.

Adjusting

I would hope by now you're also starting to notice changes in your appetite and have an adjusted view on food.

For example, you should now realize that the calorie cost of an appetizer, entrée and a desert, is not outweighed by eating a salad with tons of veggies.

Eating "healthy" isn't really the same as eating less. Eating more than your daily calorie goal worth of healthy foods will still result in weight gain.

Losing weight and eating healthy don't really mean the same thing. Over eating leads to weight gain. Where you're getting the calories from doesn't affect your body weight, however this isn't a free pass to eat junk food.

Like I said earlier, junk food doesn't keep you keep full so yes, you'll still lose weight; but eating poorly will probably just lead to other health problems.

Take the time to scroll through the days you've already logged your food for and take note of where you're spending the most. As you shed pounds, assuming you update your current weight, your tracking app will recalculate how many calories you can eat per day.

So, for example you may be able to eat 2300 calories per day and still lose a pound per week. After you've lost 5 pounds or so you'll notice that the app will update and you can now only have 2000 calories per day.

Of course, those are just example numbers and real numbers will vary person to person but the concept is the same; the more you lose, the less you have to lose. Your appetite should adjust to account for your new eating habits so don't feel like it's a permanent uphill battle.

Once you have reached your goal weight you will slowly establish this as your natural resting point. Your weight may vary occasionally but as long as you stay on top of it, bouncing back shouldn't be an issue.

Tracking your weight loss really is as simple as monitoring calories taken in and weight/neck/hips/waist measuring.

You're probably starting to feel pretty enlightened by now as you've cleared your mind of all the nonsense and misinformation that the media has spread to so many people; convincing them that they need to take nine different pills and powders to achieve their fitness goals.

Having clear goals in sight and knowing that what you are doing is the only way to meet your goals makes it that much more critically important and that much easier to stay motivated and keep on track.

Don't worry about nonsense claims that there is an alternative to eating within your calorie goal and working hard to achieve your fitness goals.

The motivation that comes from seeing your body transform over a period of time is euphoric. It's an excellent lesson in learning that good things take time and cannot be rushed.

Just keep on pushing forward every day and soon it will all seem like it wasn't even a big deal. Patience is key and learning how to wait for things worth waiting for is a lesson everyone can benefit from. You just have to trust that good things will come from hard work and dedication.

The gym is also an excellent place to have some time to yourself.

Load up your favourite songs onto your phone/mp3 player, put on some decent headphones and let the time pass while you lift and focus. It can actually be very stress relieving and with great results to boot! Nothing quite compares to getting a new one rep max while listening to your favourite workout song.

Others who are considering purchasing this book would love to know what you think. If you could spare a few seconds, they would greatly appreciate reading an honest review from you. Simply visit the page on Amazon.com.

The Final Push

Dieting Week 3

21 days of dieting and going strong I hope. If you find yourself still fighting your appetite, water and vegetables are your new best friend. Vegetables are cheap, low in calories, are good for you (obviously) and keep you feeling full.

Same goes for chicken and rice, in fact many weightlifters are familiar with an unseasoned chicken breast with a side of rice and steamed vegetables. It may seem like a pretty bland meal but it's quick, cheap, and anybody can whip it together in the kitchen.

Having a lackluster meal sure beats going to bed knowing that you overate that day.

If you absolutely need a snack in between meals, look no further than your local grocery store. "Healthy" snack foods are somewhat trendy and have grown in popularity.

If you must snack, don't blow your calories on cheese puffs and soft drinks, spend it on things like Veggie Straws.

Snacks like Veggie Straws are not terrible for you but most importantly have a large serving size and are low in calories.

Obviously, carrots and a glass of water is ideal but sometimes you just have to snack and already burned up your cheat day.

This is when a bag of low calorie snack food and some diet soft drink can save the day. Just stroll down the snack food aisle and lookout for anything that looks remotely decent.

Sooner or later your cravings for salty junk food and sugary drinks will degrade to the point where you honestly don't even joy them anymore. This is pretty a much as big of a sign of a changing appetite as you're going to get. You learn new recipes, cook smaller portions, and push junk further and further out of your diet.

The worst thing you can do while dieting and tracking calories, is to slack off. Once you start "forgetting" to track that granola bar or glass of orange juice is when you start to give up.

If you've been tracking your calories for any decent length of time, you won't give up all at once, you'll start to neglect adding the odd food item.

Soon you'll start skipping entire meal logs and eventually entire days up until the point where your tracking app just sits on your home screen, unused.

The best way to stop digging this hole is to stop it from growing in the first place. Make it a point of your day that you will sit down sometime and make sure every single thing you ate that day gets logged.

You can cheat your tracking app, but your body can't cheat away those calories.

Dieting

Dieting is the most honest thing because there simply are no cutting corners. There are calories in and calories out.

You can try to convince yourself otherwise, you may even succeed, but in the end, you cannot bargain with weight loss, you cannot cheat weight loss and you cannot trick weight loss. There is only tracking, patience and dedication.

Meal replacement shakes another option you could explore. They aren't the most affordable option but there are websites that compare the dollar per scoop for different brands and tell you which the best buy is at the time. These are great if you don't want to plan and prep your breakfast or lunch.

Just mix the serving size with water or milk (the package says mix with your favorite beverage but the only good experiences I've had was with milk or water) and scan the barcode. Super simple solution if you're lazy or just don't have the time.

The down side to these shakes is that they aren't exactly the most filling thing to eat.

There are also appetite suppressant pills but these seem questionable to me. I would only ever try these if you're desperate to get your appetite under control and only after you talk to your family doctor about using them. They'll probably ask to see the ingredient list.

Instead of buying a bottle and then finding out you can't take them, look for the product on bodybuilding.com and you can see the nutritional label and ingredient list online. Show them on your phone and take their advice; you won't find somebody with better advice for your health than a doctor.

The supplements I have used only ever seemed to have very limited effects and often upset my stomach to the point where it interfered with my workout.

I advise against using them because I think they are a waste of money and even if they do help you lose weight, is it really worth the risks? Will you have to keep taking these suppressants to stop yourself from bouncing back to overeating?

Exercising Week 3

There are usually variations you can perform for exercises if you feel like mixing it up.

For example, I like to use the leg sled machine (sometimes called leg press) with both legs and about 4 sets of 5-8 reps and then take a short break before doing one leg presses. It's similar enough that you can jump right into and are already warmed up but different enough that you really feel the muscle engagement.

As I mentioned earlier, you have your warm up set and you're working sets. Your warmup set is typically performed with a weight that you can lift with ease.

Your goal is to get into the proper motions and mindset. Feel your muscles contract at the peak of the lift. Watch your form in the mirror and make sure that your working sets have the same good form as your warm up set.

As for your working sets, I recommend finding out what your 1 rep max is, and then lifting about 80% - 90% of that number. So, if you can bench 150lbs for 1 rep, you're working sets should be anywhere from 120lbs to 135 for 5-8 reps, 3-4 working sets.

For example, warm up with 115lbs for 8 reps, then proceed with your working sets. Start off with at least 80% or 120lbs for 5 reps and at most 135lbs for 8 reps.

If you feel that you easily lift 135 for more than 8 reps, it is time to attempt a new 1 rep max. Add weight slowly and always use a spotter, especially when attempting to lift a new max.

This applies mostly for the big lifts, like squats, deadlifts and bench. You won't typically see people attempting a 1 rep max for arm curls or triceps extensions. Probably because these are smaller muscle groups and are easier to damage with heavy weight.

Do's and Don'ts

Another thing to note is that you may have sloppy form when first starting off lifting. Don't worry about this, as with more practice comes more stable form. You just need to give your body some time to adjust to these new movements, especially if you've had a rather sedentary life prior.

Just don't push yourself with heavy weight until you've got a solid lifting foundation. You'll get this from watching video guides either on bodybuilding.com or YouTube and then watching yourself perform the lifts in the mirror and mentally comparing yourself to the video.

Keep an eye out for the quality of the instructions though. 10 likes and 500 dislikes? Find another instructional video to watch. People are quick to criticize inaccurate information on the internet, and you certainly don't want to take bad lifting advice. You only get one body, take care of it!

The most common form flaws I've noticed are: swinging the weight for arm curls, excessively bouncing the weight off the chest for bench press, leaning too far forwards for squats, and bouncing the weight off the floor for deadlifts.

To avoid these mistakes let's go through them one at a time. When performing an arm curl, your forearm should be the only thing that's moving. Watch yourself in the mirror and see if your elbow is moving, or if you're leaning back to assist the lift.

When performing bench press, I've seen some people literally bounce the weight off their chest to build up some momentum to drive the weight upwards. Don't do this for obvious reasons. The weight should, at most, touch your chest.

It's often debated whether or not your back should lift up at all, or whether bringing the weight all the way to touch your chest is correct. My argument would be to try things not set in stone and do what's most comfortable for your specific body type.

When performing squats, it's surprisingly easy to lean too far forwards. You'll know you're leaning too far forwards if you're using the front half of your foot and toes to keep yourself balanced. The weight should be mostly on your heels.

When performing deadlifts, the weight should reach a full stop in between lifts. Hence the name, deadlift, as in lifting dead weight. There should be a slight pause after the weight is back on the floor. You don't want to build momentum. Think of it like starting the lift over for every rep.

Another point about deadlifts, lifting louder is not a substitute for lifting correctly. The weight coming down should not be loud at all. This indicates a lack of control over the weight.

Finishing your Workout

Let's talk about lifting until failure, just so you know what people are talking about if they mention it. Lifting until failure is exactly what it sounds like.

Perform the exercise until you can no longer perform any reps at all. If you plan on doing this, save it for the end of your workout.

Take a break after you've performed all your exercises for that muscle group for the day and then pick an exercise to perform until failure (I would limit lifting until failure to one exercise), and lift that weight until you cannot continue. Personally, I prefer to combine this concept with drop sets (burn sets).

Drop sets are performed by starting off with the heaviest weight you can perform the lift with and lifting until failure. Then you set that weight back on the rack and drop the weight by about

10lbs and immediately start lifting again until failure with no break.

Drop the weight by 5-10 pounds again and repeat. Drop again by another 5lbs and lift until failure and you've now completed a drop set. Needless to say, this is considered a finisher and is reserved as the last part of your workout.

A finisher is just slang for an exercise that is preferred to end off a workout with.

The reason they are preferred for finishing a workout is because they are simple movements that don't take a ton of energy to perform but you can really feel your already worked muscles get that last level of engagement.

My favourite finishers are: drop set of arm curls for biceps, drop set of standing triceps extensions, push-ups for chest/triceps, planking for abs, dips for chest/triceps, cable rows for middle back, chin-ups for upper back, dumbbell shrugs for upper back, standing calf raises and one leg presses on the leg sled.

That should be enough advice to get you started lifting safely and correctly. Make this the beginning of a new, healthier lifestyle. There are so many benefits to weightlifting, the people you meet, the personal goals you set and achieve for yourself and the all the health benefits that follow.

I would go so far as to say that everybody, barring those with pre-existing medical conditions and injuries, should look into weightlifting and strength training.

Results Week 3

I hope you took a starting picture to compare your results with. It validates all of the hard work you put in to get these results.

If you are starting to see results, the considered healthy range would be somewhere between 1.5lbs to 6lbs lost in three weeks.

This is based on three weeks times the weight loss goals MyFitnessPal allows you to choose. Whether you chose the goal of 0.5lbs per week or 2lbs per week, or somewhere in between, just know what you're doing is worth it.

I should also mention that which lbs/week weight loss goal you chose directly affects how many calories per day you can eat.

Want to lose more weight? Consume fewer calories. Were you a little too ambitious with your choice? Eat more calories but know that your results will come slower.

You may find that in the coming weeks you have to tweak you profile and make some adjusts.

Another tip here to help you avoid midnight snacks: brush your teeth. When you've already eaten up all of your calories for the day, one more snack before bed can be tempting.

The best way to crush this is to brush your teeth, floss and head to bed. Now you know if you get up and have that last piece of ice cream birthday cake in the fridge, not only did you go over your limit for the day, now you have to brush and floss all over again. Not to mention minty toothpaste mouth can turn any tasty snack pretty nasty.

Final Things To Keep In Mind

Keep in mind that the absolute fewest calories an adult male can consume per day is 1500 calories and 1200 for females. These are the bottom numbers and for people who have no physical activity in the day.

This would result in extreme weight loss overtime when people do this extreme dieting, it often results in bouncing right back to their starting weight. The reason for this is because your body never had a chance to adjust. Your appetite will be going crazy and you can only fight it for so long. You have to do weight loss in a controlled manner and do it over weeks and months.

Maybe you could even use these fitness results as motivation way to kick an unhealthy habit, like smoking.

If you're a long-time smoker, you'll notice the effects it has on you while trying to become fit. Shortness of breath sound familiar? After some time exercising, you're sure to get better stamina, especially if you chose to run.

Get addicted to running instead of cigarettes. If you feel strongly enough about running you'll kick smoking, not because they're bad for you, but because they are holding you back from reaching that new running goal.

Keep in mind smoking will hold back all of your fitness results to some degree, same with excessive alcohol intake. You'll be more tired and more easily winded.

If you want the absolute best results possible, you'll need to kick more than just the habit of overeating.

Never lose sight of the true end goal here. The final result you're trying to achieve here. A healthier, more active you. Whether you lose 10lbs in the next two months by cutting out deserts and playing catch with your dog or becoming the next bodybuilding icon lifting record amounts of weight, know that what you did was for the betterment of yourself.

The degree to which you went is arbitrary. After all, you set the goal. I hope that there is enough here to get you kick started on a path towards that goal. The only person who can reach this goal, is you.

I hope you have learned something from this book so far and would greatly appreciate it if you could leave an honest review on Amazon.com.

Are You ALWAYS Hungry When You Try to Lose Weight?

Discover How to STOP Starving Yourself & Lose Weight FASTER By Eating MORE Food!

For this month only, you can get Kayla's best-selling & most popular book absolutely free – *The Ultimate Guide to Healthy Eating & Losing Weight Without Starving Yourself!*

Get Your FREE Copy Here:
TopFitnessAdvice.com/Book

Discover how you can **start eating MORE food** and see weight loss results faster than ever before. Learn about the 10 most powerful fat-burning foods and how they boost the rate that your body burns fat. And last but not least, finally put an end to your emotional or "bored" eating habits. With this book, readers were able to significantly improve their weight loss results. So, it's highly recommended that you get this book, especially while it's free!

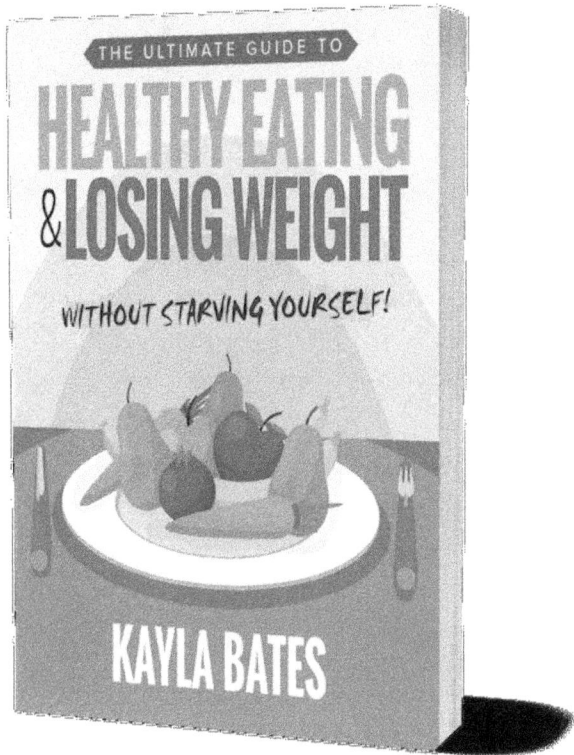

THE ULTIMATE GUIDE TO

HEALTHY EATING & LOSING WEIGHT

WITHOUT STARVING YOURSELF!

KAYLA BATES

Get Your FREE Copy Here:

TopFitnessAdvice.com/Book

Conclusion

So, let's summarize what we've learned here today. Eating fewer calories is the core of weight loss and it does not demand that you sacrifice your favorite foods or give up nights out on the town with your friends.

We learned that you can still eat fast food and that restaurants are not your enemy. We learned that even multiple ingredient home cooked meals can still be logged.

We've learned that working out doesn't magically transform fat into muscles, really what happens is that you are burning fat reserves and adding muscle mass.

We learned that the only reason people believe in fitness shortcuts is because it's more comforting to imagine that you just haven't found the right magic pill than to acknowledge the only way to good fitness is diet and exercise.

Another myth dispelled was that you need to run on the treadmill to lose weight. Not only is cardio not mandatory for weight loss, I actually find it makes it more difficult as it can increase your appetite.

We went over some starting exercises like the bench press, squat and deadlift. We learned how to put together a basic exercise schedule. We learned that crunches, the smith machine and leg extensions should be ejected from anyone's workout routine and replaced with planking, free weights and the leg press.

Also covered was a few basic variations on popular exercise, like leg press vs. one leg presses.

Another key point covered was that your first set is considered your warm up set and the 3-4 sets after that are considered working sets.

Remember that working sets should be about 80% - 90% of your one rep max. We also covered how to record your lifts and the significance of doing so.

Also, a good rep range to stick to is 5-8. If you can easily lift 90% for more than 8 reps, its time to go up in weight. Maybe attempt a new one rep max?

We went through drop sets and finishers and explained what they are and how to do them. We talked about what their purpose is and what exercises are good to perform them for.

A crucial point of dieting, record every piece of food you consume. Logging your meals is unavoidable when it comes to weight loss. You have to know your calorie goal based on age, height, gender, current weight and activity level, and update your weight as you make progress.

We learned about progress pictures and how to connect them with the associated body weight in our tracking app. We also covered why they are important and how they serve to motivate you to stay in shape once you get there.

We spoke briefly on common mistakes for popular exercises, how to identify them and how to avoid them. We looked at some different sources for checking form and discovering new exercises/alternative method, YouTube and bobybuilding.com being your new best friends.

Another point mentioned is how important it is to have you own time and space to unwind after a long day at work and the gym can be that place.

It doesn't have to be the gym necessarily but as long you can listen to your favourite workout music and get some good exercise done in the day, it really will help you unwind unlike anything else. It's even good for you to boot!

I've already said this but I'm going to say it again, because I think it's the most important thing I have to say. Know that what you are doing, regardless of the results, is in an attempt to try and better yourself.

There are no fitness goals besides the ones that you set for yourself. There will always be somebody faster than you, and stronger than you. You were never meant to compare yourself to other people. The only comparison that really matters in fitness, is comparing the current you to the old you.

Best of luck in the adventure that is life and do the best you can to stay fit and stay healthy.

Don't forget to share your thoughts on this book by leaving a review on Amazon.com. It takes just a few seconds.

Enjoying this book?

Check out my other best sellers!

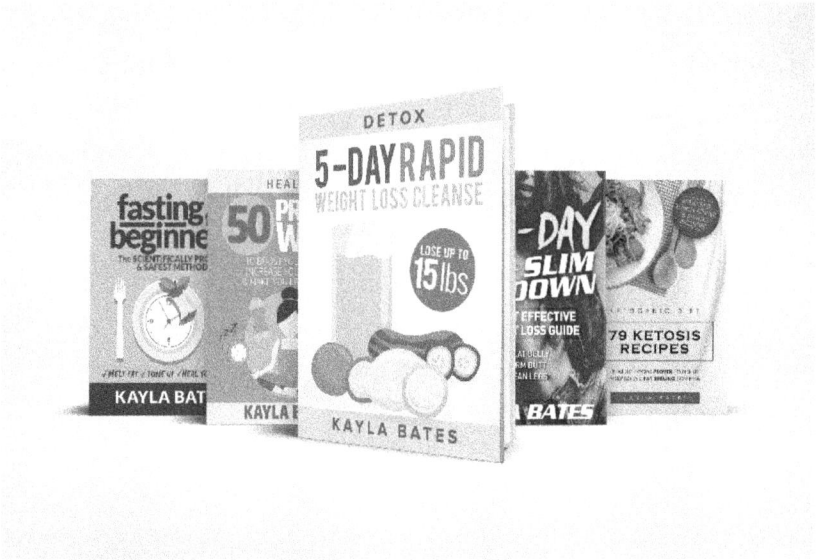

Final Words

I would like to thank you for purchasing my book and I hope I have been able to help you and educate you on something new.

If you have enjoyed this book and would like to share your positive thoughts, could you please take 30 seconds of your time to go back and give me a review on my Amazon book page.

I greatly appreciate seeing these reviews because it helps me share my hard work.

You can leave me a review on Amazon.com.

Again, thank you and I wish you all the best!

www.ingramcontent.com/pod-product-compliance
Lightning Source LLC
Chambersburg PA
CBHW031206020426
42333CB00013B/816